The Last Blessing

The Last Blessing

Every Life is a story..
Every story has a Blessing

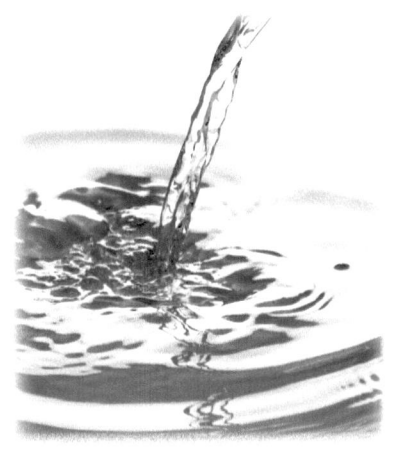

Michelle Poston,
Ronald Lewis

Xulon Elite

Xulon Press
2301 Lucien Way #415
Maitland, FL 32751
407.339.4217
www.xulonpress.com

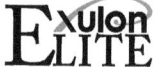

© 2017 by Michelle Poston, Ronald Lewis

All rights reserved solely by the author. The author guarantees all contents are original and do not infringe upon the legal rights of any other person or work. No part of this book may be reproduced in any form without the permission of the author. The views expressed in this book are not necessarily those of the publisher.

Scripture quotations taken from the King James Version (KJV) – *public domain*.

Hymn taken from The Celebration Hymnal. Copyright 1997 by Word Music.

Edited by Xulon Press.

Printed in the United States of America.

ISBN-13: 9781545615300

Dedication

We dedicate *The Last Blessing* to our Lord Jesus Christ and thank Him for giving us His inspiration and the gift to write. This book is a testimony of all who have died and all who have lived and received the promised blessings of God's Holy and divine Word. We thank God for His grace and mercy in allowing us to work in the demanding and difficult field of hospice. Most of all, we thank God for His forgiveness and Salvation through Jesus Christ.

We have both been through many difficult times, but God has granted us the strength to endure. This life is just a stopping place and only for a moment. The prize is heaven and eternal life.

Colossians 3:17 "Whatever you do in word or deed, do all in the name of the Lord Jesus, giving thanks through Him to God the Father."

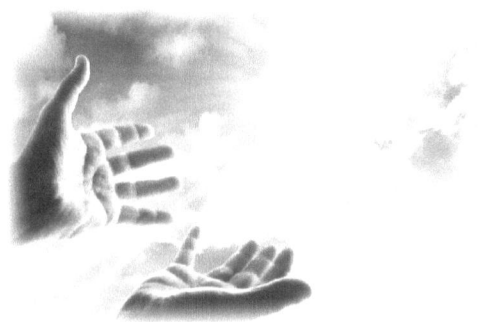

The Last Blessing

Every life is a story, and every story has a blessing

By Michelle Poston, RN
Ronald Lewis, Chaplain

As an outreach ministry of

The Poston Russ Foundation

Spreading God's Simple Plan for Salvation

Proverbs 14:31 "Whoever oppresses a poor man insults his maker, but he who is generous to the needy honors him."

A Non-Profit Organization

In Loving Memory of Zanny Poston, Eva Mae Poston, John Russ, and Catherine Russ

Preface

Every life is a story, and every story has a blessing.

The Last Blessing is a compilation of real-life stories about our experience in witnessing God's presence and blessings upon those diagnosed with terminal illnesses.

It was written to spiritually empower patients, caregivers, and families during the most difficult time in their lives. *The Last Blessing* reveals God's unchanging love, forgiveness, and gift of Salvation unto all who seek Him.

Table of Contents

Introduction xv

Chapter 1 - Hospice 1
Chapter 2 - Hope 3
Chapter 3 - Heaven Can Wait 7
Chapter 4 - First Death 11
Chapter 5 - Symptom Management 15
Chapter 6 - Home/Homeless to Home 27
Chapter 7 - Forgiven 31
Chapter 8 - Timesharing 35
Chapter 9 - Alzheimer's 37
Chapter 10 - Go Tigers 45
Chapter 11 - Grief 47
Chapter 12 - A Change of Mind 53

Conclusion 57
Hymn-Amazing Grace 59
Reference 61
Resources 63
About the Authors 65

Introduction

Written by Michelle
The Last Blessing was born on April 24, 2017. This is an account of the events of that day:

Hospice was not an easy job, so our hospice team would meet first thing on Monday mornings to go over the events of the weekend and changes in policy, as well as to get on the same page to better help our patients. Chaplain Ron started the meeting with prayer requests and our weekly devotion. The topic of devotion was taken from Deuteronomy 23:21-23 and basically states we must keep any promises and vows that we make.

We were all in our seats and I was trying to get online to work on my notes for the Wednesday Interdisciplinary meeting, where we discuss each patient and their needs. Everyone was online working diligently except for me. I couldn't get online. I asked several people to look at my computer, but no one could figure out why I could not get online. I had a deadline; I had not finished the previous week's documentation, and I was going to be in trouble, not to mention I had to also work on my interdisciplinary group meeting notes. I grew increasingly anxious. I started having sharp pains in my stomach and abdomen. *I have got to get out of here.* The pain grew sharper and more intense.

Finally, two hours later, the meeting was over. Chaplain Ron came over and asked, "Hey Michelle, is everything okay?"

I was pale and sick, I replied, "I will call you later."

He replied, "Okay, I will talk to you later; don't forget about lunch."

In a few hours, I felt a little better, so I decided to meet Chaplain Ron for pizza. During our lunch, I said, "I feel something isn't right." He assured me, as he had many times, this was Satan trying to discourage me. At that moment, out of left field, I had a crazy thought. "Ron," I said, "I believe we need to write a book together: *The Tale of Death*.

He looked at me oddly and said, "What did you say? Say that again."

"*The Tale of Death*, no, *The Face of Death*. Ron, I believe God wants us to write a book about our experiences in hospice. I see my grandmother's masked face as she was dying." *I am going crazy*, I thought; I was literally seeing dead people. I believe Ron thought I was going crazy too.

"Really, Michelle! I don't know." He looked at me as if I had two heads, but we started talking about our experiences and how many people God had blessed during the most critical time in their lives. We realized that through God's inspiration and direction, we could help many people: people diagnosed with a terminal illness, family members who don't know what to expect, caregivers who have to carry the burden of care alone, and healthcare professionals would all benefit from our experiences.

At 5:00 pm I was happy to be home, but sad because I was on-call. The scrubs came off and I was in my favorite sweatshirt and pants. Being a hospice nurse had many ups and many downs, and call was a down. Most people believe being with a dying patient is the worst part of the job. Believe it or not, death was not the worst part. For me, the worst part was call. I hated call. I loathed call. I despised call. I could work all day and if I got a call, I could end up working all night and have to work the next day. The company I worked for paid a nurse to take call, but it wasn't enough to warrant working all day and all night. My life literally stopped while I was on-call. It can be described as a sitting duck waiting to be shot.

The phone rang around 9:00 pm. A patient's urinary catheter was leaking, which is not something that could be taken care of by phone. I thought to myself, *I bet his catheter is not leaking*. I was aggravated and I had a bad attitude. I was tired and needed to complete the charts for the patients I had assessed earlier that day. I was very far behind on my documentation and my work was far from over, but the scrubs came back on and I was on the road again.

I drove thirty miles to a little town. When I turned off the main road onto a back road, the sky got darker. I drove slowly and found the little home surrounded by trees and woods. I knocked on the door and an elderly lady opened the door. She was stooped over and unable to stand straight. "I'm sorry," she said. "I feel bad you had to come all this way, but I didn't know what to do." She truly felt bad for me. I walked into the home and was surrounded by clutter. In all my years of visiting patients I had seen many cluttered homes, but this one took the cake. I walked into the den and there was a recliner with a small television in the middle of the room. The couch was surrounded by boxes, toys, mountains of clothes, and a few old televisions. The den was open to the kitchen. There was no table in the kitchen, only boxes. There was a narrow path to walk through the home. The home may have been around eight hundred square feet, but had enough stuff to fill a mansion. Some spots had boxes from the floor to the ceiling.

I followed the path down the middle of the hallway. At the end of the hallway was a bathroom. Through the open door I could see the tub was full of clothes and boxes that reached from the bottom of the tub to the ceiling. *Where do you bathe?* I thought. There was only one bathroom, but I did not ask; I kept my mouth shut.

Through the clutter, I found the patient in a bedroom. It was a tiny room with a hospital bed, a single bed, and boxes from the floor to the ceiling. *How sweet,* I thought, *She sleeps beside him every night.* The patient was obese and confused. The room smelt of urine and the bed was filled with urine soaked towels. The wife was correct; the urinary catheter was leaking.

I greeted him and quickly got to fixing his catheter. The patient was funny and told me wild stories of his youth. I actually enjoyed my visit and stayed about thirty minutes after I changed the catheter because he was a joy. I felt terrible because my attitude had been bad and because his catheter had needed to be changed.

Though I was enjoying the company, I was tired and ready to go home. I walked down the path to the living room. I said goodbye to the wife and asked if her husband's stories were true, to which she confirmed they were. When I opened the door to go outside, the night was cool but warm. My face felt the coolness of the night air and quickly became warm. I felt as if something was not right. As I walked down the steps toward my car, I felt very uneasy. There was no breeze and the night was eerily quiet. I was suddenly afraid—something was not right. I looked toward my car because I thought there may be an animal or person close, and I wanted to run. I thought, *should I run up the stairs and go inside and ask for help or do I run to my car.* Suddenly something told me to stop. I stood still. I was trembling. My keys were in my hand and my hand was shaking to the point I had to grip the keys tightly because I thought I was going to drop them on the dark ground. I had a tremendous feeling that I was in danger and I scanned the area. I did not see anyone or any animals. I felt as if Satan was close.

Ron told me earlier that day that Satan was going to try to stop us from writing, and that we had to stay firm and do God's will. I stood still and I felt as though I was about to be raped or attacked. I said to Satan, "If someone rapes me, I will go down praying, and I will get up and tell my testimony of how good God is. If a person or an animal kills me, I will go down praying and I will rise up in heaven. There is nothing you can do to me to stop me from serving my God."

I was terrified, but I meant every word. I calmly walked to my car, opened the door, and drove home. I felt a bad spirit, a demonic spirit. I felt as if I had just had a duel with the Devil. Ron was correct, Satan was going to try to stop God's work, but God is stronger than Satan. Good will always triumph over evil. I vowed that nothing would stop me from doing God's will.

I could barely wait till the next day to tell Chaplain Ron about what had happened. I called him bright and early. "Ron, you are not going to believe what happened last night."

I told him everything, and his words were, "Michelle, that's our confirmation from God." We knew at that moment the book was God's will and nothing would stop us. We prayed and began to write. We recalled Deuteronomy 23:21-23 and vowed that nothing would stop us from writing this book. We made a promise to each other and to God.

As we began to write and collaborate on stories, we realized that God's blessings were evident. After much prayer and consideration, (and approximately one million text messages) we decided the book should be entitled *The Last Blessing*.

Hospice

Written by Michelle

I was asked a million questions when I was a hospice nurse: What is hospice? Who pays for hospice? How do you know someone is going to die? I find most people believe hospice only takes place within a few days of the patient's death, is only for cancer patients, or is only at a Hospice House. However, hospice care can look much different than that.

I personally have a long and short definition of hospice. My long definition would be ten pages, so I will spare the long, boring definition. My short definition is end of life care for patients, their family, and caregivers in a home or facility.

There are many criteria for hospice services, such as a terminal illness with a life expectancy of six months or less, or if the patient chooses to not have or stop curative treatments.

There are many benefits to hospice. A terminal diagnosis may bring fear, uncertainty, emotional distress, and physical distress. I believe the biggest hospice benefit is the help one may receive from a team of experienced clinical professionals who understand death and the fear that a patient and caregivers may go through, and therefore can provide support.

According to the American Hospice Foundation, hospice services are paid for by Medicare (through the Hospice Benefit), Medicaid (in most states), the Veteran's Health Administration, and many private insurance companies provide some coverage for hospice care (American Hospice Foundation).

Hope

"For we are saved by hope: but hope that is seen is not hope: for what a man seeth, why doth he yet hoped for? But if we hope for that we see not, then do we with patience wait for it."
—Romans 8:24-25

Written by Michelle

Hope is a tough subject because hope has different meanings. For example, I can hope my green beans turn into ice cream, or I hope that life takes the appropriate timeline, meaning I hope that my children will outlive me. We all hope for good things in life, but what we truly hope for is a life with our loved ones.

In hospice, we define hope as trust. We trust that our patients will be pain free, trust that we will manage all symptoms, and trust that all needs will be met, including the caregiver's needs.

Many times, people lose control when they are diagnosed with a terminal illness, and people can become hopeless when they lose control. Hopelessness is equivalent to being in a dark hole. Hope has light. Hope has life. Even a dying person can have hope—hope for eternal life, hope of seeing their deceased loved ones in heaven, hope that their loved ones on earth will be taken care of, and hope to make the best of every day.

I learned a long time ago not to take away hope. Without hope one cannot survive. I never lied to my patients, but I did not always give all the information. If I was asked questions, I tried to be honest without taking away hope.

The following are two stories where I tried to keep hope alive.

We received a referral for a sixty-year-old male with pancreatic cancer. I arrived at his beautiful home outside of town the day after he was diagnosed. I learned this patient had never been sick and started feeling bad a few weeks before. He saw a doctor and after a few tests, was diagnosed. The patient's wife said, "The doctor walked in the room and said you have pancreatic cancer and you have two weeks to live. He walked out the room without saying another word." They were in shock to say the least. The doctor in essence took away all hope from this man.

I did my physical assessment, read over the lab values and the doctor's report. His cancer was too advanced for treatment. My grandmother died of pancreatic cancer, so this case was like pouring salt into a wound. Many memories came pouring in and I thought, *How can I do this?* I did not want to remember the sad memories, but as the assessment progressed, I continued to remember. One day my grandmother was working in her garden and being the best mother and grandmother in the world, the next week she was in bed sick, the following week she was diagnosed with pancreatic cancer, and the next week she was in a hospital bed dying.

The wife asked to see me in private and we walked toward the sunroom. The sunroom had been built by himself with his own tools. As I walked, my legs were heavy, very heavy. She had quietly cried through the assessment, and I knew she was upset and wanted answers. I wanted to run out the door; I did not want to go into that room. I was upset that this lovely couple was about to have their lives turned upside down. I was also remembering the pain from my grandmother's death. *I can't do this,* was all I could think. I just wanted to leave.

Inside the sunroom, I was a cornered animal. I couldn't have gotten out if I had tried. I was stuck. The sweet lady burst into tears and asked, "How many people survive pancreatic cancer? Why won't the doctor allow us to try radiation or chemo? Is there any chance we could see another doctor and have chemo or radiation? Should we get a second opinion? What can he do to live longer than two weeks? How many of your patients have survived pancreatic cancer?"

I could not give her an answer, because I would have taken everything from her. I was trying to hold back my tears. I was thinking of a way to tell her the truth without taking away her hope. I am sure I looked like a deer in headlights. She looked at me with tears in her eyes and I could see that she wanted to scream, "Answer me!" She did not scream, but she sweetly said, "Help me."

I wanted to run. I really wanted to run. I did not want to be there; I did not want to live through this. I was an adult when my grandmother died, and I remembered asking the same questions. I calmly said, "God is in control. God's will will be done." I explained that I had witnessed many patients with a terminal diagnosis who were blessed to live longer than their diagnosis-expectancy.

The patient was sick at times, but was not in pain and overall had mild symptoms. I explained that she and her husband should try to stay positive and continue with their normal routine. I wanted them to enjoy time with their grandchildren and friends. I encouraged her to try not to concentrate on the diagnosis, but to concentrate on enjoying every moment that he was not sick. She wiped her eyes and with a sweet country accent she said, "thank you". She accepted my response and did not push me any further. She knew what I was saying even though I did not say it.

The patient and his wife took my advice and tried to stay positive. The next four weeks were mostly spent at church, the beach, the park, and the zoo. The patient spent most of his time living and only spent the last few days in bed. He had good days and bad days, but most of his days were good. I honestly believe if I had taken away their hope, the patient would have spent those four weeks in bed dying.

I once had an elderly patient. He was bedbound, his kidneys were shutting down, and he was dying. His poor wife wanted him to live. She was a wonderful wife and caregiver, and she couldn't bear life without him. She could barely take care of herself, but she took wonderful care of this man. She took care of her husband better than she took care of herself.

One day she looked me in the eye and told me her husband's driver's license was about to expire. She wanted to schedule transport to take him to the DMV to get his license renewed. I looked at her and expected her to start laughing. She did not laugh. I was respectfully laughing on the inside while I waited on her to give the punch line. She was serious. I was in disbelief. This woman was not demented, she was very much mentally stable. She knew her husband was dying, and she knew her husband was in hospice care. I was dumbfounded. My mind was racing, trying to figure out how this man could possibly get out of a bed and walk, let alone drive. My mind wandered to a vision: I could see myself telling my supervisor that we were paying for transport for a dying patient to go to the DMV to get his license renewed. I could see myself being fired—trust me, I would have gotten fired. I could see the patient on a stretcher rolling into the DMV. When it was clear that she was serious, I said, "I don't believe your husband is able to drive at this time and I feel we should wait to call transport." That was a difficult conversation, I could not call transport and I couldn't take away her hope. She was a Christian woman and she was surrounded with family and friends. When her husband went to heaven, she was accepting. She knew her husband was in heaven and she knew she would see him again.

I had a great loss in my life and I found peace in Hebrews 6:19 "Which hope we have as an anchor of the soul, both sure and stedfast, and which entereth into that within the veil." It has been my experience that hope is an anchor and a requirement for those that are living and for those that are dying.

Heaven Can Wait

In those days was Hezekiah sick unto death. And Isaiah the prophet the son of Amoz came unto him, and said unto him, Thus saith the LORD, Set thine house in order: for thou shalt die, and not live.
Then Hezekiah turned his face toward the wall, and prayed unto the LORD,
And said, Remember now, O LORD, I beseech thee, how I have walked before thee in truth and with a perfect heart, and have done that which is good in thy sight. And Hezekiah wept sore.
Then came the word of the LORD to Isaiah, saying, Go, and say to Hezekiah, Thus saith the LORD, the God of David thy father, I have heard thy prayer, I have seen thy tears: behold, I will add unto thy days fifteen years.

—Isaiah 38:1-5

Written by Michelle

One of my patients was diagnosed with cancer twelve years previously. He was given a death sentence, but survived the odds. The man was a son, husband, and father. He was very religious and claimed Jesus Christ as his Lord and Savior.

Unfortunately, the cancer came back and once again he was admitted to hospice with a poor prognosis. His family was positive and felt God would spare is life a second time. We had many talks about God and their faith. Twelve years was a long time and I told the family he was a walking miracle. He had twelve years to do all the things he had not done previously. He and his family went on many vacations, he finished all the projects he wanted to finish around the house. He was at the hospital with his children when his grandchildren were born, and he enjoyed their early years. He volunteered in his church and helped everyone in his neighborhood.

I met multiple family, friends, and church members. You could see the love everyone had for this man. His wife was distraught beyond words. One of my sweetest memories as a hospice nurse was walking into this tiny house and seeing the patient in his hospital bed in the middle of the living room. His wife was seated in a chair next to the bed, and the room was full of friends from their church. They made a big circle while holding hands around the perimeter of the room and prayed. I walked into the room and held the wife's hand and prayed with everyone. It was very touching to see their love and faith.

Unfortunately, the patient got weaker and weaker. A few days later I heard his wife stand over her husband's bed and beg him not to die. "I can't live without you," she sobbed, "and you told my mother you would take care of me." As the end grew near, we discussed death and a life without her husband. She understood God was going to take her husband, and she came to terms with his fate. She thanked God for the gift of twelve years. The patient was blessed to die pain free in his home, with his family and church friends at his bedside. I call this story bittersweet. He had a wonderful life, and his family was devastated and would surely miss this wonderful man. The sweet side is better than the bitter side because this man was in heaven. There was no doubt where he was and there was no doubt his family would see him again in heaven.

Words For Thought From Chaplain Ron

A diagnosis of a terminal illness does not necessarily mean that one will face death according to a prescribed timeline, because each and every one of our lives is in the hands of God. This case reminded me of the story of King Hezekiah found in Isaiah 38:1-5. God sent Isaiah to tell the king to get his house in order because he would soon die. However, after the king wept and prayed, God sent Isaiah back to let him know that his prayers had been heard, his tears had been seen, and that God had added fifteen more years to his life.

Be encouraged and never give up hope. Embrace each and every day that God gives with thanksgiving. For although you or a loved one may have been given a prognosis as such in this case, God may be saying, *heaven can wait*!

The First Death

Blessed are those who mourn, for they will be comforted.
—Matthew 5:4

Written by Michelle

In nursing school, I was taught how to help patients to live and avoid death. When a nurse works in a facility, she usually works three days per week, goes to work at 7:00 am, and works diligently to take care of her patients till 7:00 pm. The nurse leaves work and goes home to her life. My first nursing experience dealing with death was not pleasant, but I was not devastated. The patient was in a facility, and I had only seen the patient a few times. I had training on what to expect when a patient dies and this death did not upset me. My first hospice death, however, was not easy. I was very involved with the patient and her family. I was too involved. Hospice was new to me, and I did not know how to be a hospice nurse.

Being a hospice nurse is different. You see your patients and their loved ones at least once per week, and many times your visits are in their home. As the patient declines, the visits increase. It is very easy to weave yourself into the patient's life.

My first hospice death was a cancer patient. She lived about twenty minutes from my home and she and her family were very needy—they worried over everything. The first time the husband called after hours, Marie was on-call and he was very upset. "Marie," he screamed, "you are not my nurse, I need to talk to

Michelle." After that, I gave him my personal cell number. He called night and day and I was more than eager to accept the calls and make extra visits. I was enjoying taking care of the patient, and I was also enjoying the fact that they needed me. I felt as if I was making a difference in this patient's life.

Through the months, the patient continued to decline, and I offered nursing support, emotional support, and family support. I was working forty hours per week seeing other patients, working too many hours with this patient, and working as a mom and wife.

My daughter was in a dance company and a trip to Disney World was planned. Her company was invited to perform at Disney. I was such a good nurse, so I thought, that I planned for the patient to die when I returned from Disney. I was *sure* she would not die while I was away. I had worked hard and I believed God was going to allow her death to wait till I returned home. On the morning we were leaving, I had the car and children packed and ready to go, but I could not leave without seeing my patient. I will never forget how upset my children and husband were. They were excited and ready to leave and all I wanted to do was take care of my patient.

My husband said, "There are other nurses and you are off today, why are you going to work?" We left for Disney after a quick visit to check on my patient. One thing I learned that day, you don't keep two children waiting to go to Disney. It was not a pleasant ride. Everyone was upset, especially me. I did not want to leave my patient.

As my husband drove all day, I watched my phone. The nurses I worked with had been instructed to call me with any changes on this patient. I received no calls, so I was relieved. After unloading the car at the hotel, I called the on-call nurse to check in. "Michelle," she said, "I'm sorry, but she died earlier today."

I was devastated. "Why did you not call me?" I asked over and over. The nurse explained that there was nothing I could do, and she wanted me to have a safe trip. I hung up and called the patient's husband. He had a spirit in his voice. He loved his wife beyond what God required; he fought and did everything he could to keep her alive. He gave her everything she needed. Now it was over. I was crushed and I wept. This was not my family, but I was crying to the point I could not talk. The husband was comforting me. This was wrong. I should have been comforting him. He thanked me for all I had done.

"Don't ever doubt that you are a good nurse," he said. I could hear the strength in his voice, and I knew he was going to be okay. I will never forget his words; they were like honey to my soul. He was correct. I was a good nurse, and I did a great job.

I put my disappointment and frustration aside, and my family and I had a good trip.

I think of this wonderful family often, and I learned much from this case. A nurse can't tie herself into the lives of her patients. It is not healthy. A nurse won't be a nurse for long if she is unable to put distance between herself and her patients.

Written by Chaplain Ron

It is very difficult to not get attached to patients and their families, especially when they are on hospice services sometimes for many years. While driving down the highway one day, I remembered my first hospice patient who had passed away, and before I knew it, tears were running down my face. It's tough for me sometimes, but thank God for heaven and salvation through Jesus Christ. For as I remember my first death and others, I have said it more times than once, if they could speak to me now, I believe they would tell me, "It is well with my soul."

Symptom Management

Written by Michelle

Decreased Appetite

When my children ask me to cook something, I am on cloud nine and over the moon happy. I have always tried to cook every dish my children and friends request. One day my son asked me to cook ham and rice, and my daughter asked me to cook chicken and rice. I cooked all day that Saturday, and it was worth every second to see them eat something they each wanted.

As a society, our lives revolve around food. We celebrate with food, holidays revolve around food, happy hours consist of food, and we renew our relationships with family and friends over food. Food is a large part of our lives. It is this reason why patients and their families have the most difficulty dealing with decreased appetite, pain, and difficulty breathing as symptoms. When a patient is terminal and close to the end of life, he or she usually experiences a decrease in appetite. This is normal, but difficult, because family members want their loved one to eat.

There are a host of reasons why the patient might have a loss of appetite, including possible taste changes, nausea and vomiting, fear, confusion, constipation, and medication side effects. As our bodies prepare for the end, the movement in the gut slows and it is difficult to absorb fluid and nutrients. Eating food can cause diarrhea, heartburn, aspiration, and cough (verywell.com).

I had a patient who lived on liquid supplements for years because she was unable to tolerate food. Food made her sick, but she could tolerate four cans of liquid supplements per day with no gastrointestinal upset. It is a miracle in a can and provides everything a person needs to survive.

These are a few ideas that worked well with my patients with decreased appetite:

- Serve food at room temperature when possible
- Offer:
  o Non-greasy foods
  o Canned supplements and breakfast drinks are easy on the gut
  o Low fat soups, chicken broth, and beef broth
  o Crackers
  o Sorbets
  o Fruit juices
  o Soft fruits
  o Popsicles
- Offer small, frequent meals and snacks. Ensure good oral care (clean dentures and rinse mouth as often as tolerated)

I once had a patient who had breast cancer. She had a poor appetite and would barely eat. Her husband would get very upset and take her to the ER for IV fluids. Her heart was having difficulty with the IV fluids, and her upper and lower extremities would swell. The IV fluids would cause more work for her heart. Her body's organs were not working properly. God has designed our body to work a certain way. As difficult as it is, we must accept His plan.

Pain

The number one concern in hospice is pain control. I looked at every patient as if they were my father or mother, and I would not allow any patient to suffer. One of the most frustrating parts of being a hospice nurse was handling a caregiver who did not want the patient to have pain medications.

I had a patient who had dementia. She also had cardiac problems, and her legs and hands would swell. The family did not want the patient on any medications and would not allow the doctor to order medications to control her swelling. They allowed one medication for her heart, but no other medications, not even a simple OTC (over-the-counter) pain reliever. With every talk, their response was, "You don't know her; medication messes up her blood pressure." I believe the family truly believed medication would stop her heart, and I believe they loved the patient very much. The patient's extremities would swell, and the family would occasionally allow a diuretic, but only for a few days. When her extremities would swell, the patient would have terrible pain in her legs, and I would beg them to allow me to administer an OTC pain medication. They would say, "No, you don't understand what medicine does to her heart." During one visit, the patient was moaning in pain and I said to myself, "That's it." I had had it and I called our hospice physician. The physician ordered a mild prescription pain medication and a strong diuretic. He also stated, "If you find the patient moaning and in pain again, call 911." He was a wonderful doctor to work with, and he had had it too. He said, "Tell them if I make a visit to the home and the patient is in pain, I will call 911 and I will personally go with the patient to the hospital to be sure she gets clinically treated." The family allowed the medication, but only after hours of education about the patient's heart problem, why she had fluid gain, and the importance of controlling pain.

The job of hospice is to take care of a dying patient, not to try and cure a patient. We do not send a patient to the hospital; we try to manage symptoms at home. The only reason the hospice physician threated to send the patient to the hospital was because we could not allow the patient to be in pain.

I had a patient who was in his nineties and had cancer throughout his body. With this extreme presence of cancer, morphine was ordered directly after his admission and delivered to the home. The patient's wife poured the morphine down the drain and said, "That poison is not allowed in my home." There was a high probability this patient would have pain and need morphine because of his diagnosis. I begged, I pleaded, I educated; I did everything I could do, but the answer was no. She was in denial, and when she found out what hospice was, a service to help terminally ill patients with the life expectancy of six months or less, she terminated our services. I don't know what happed with this patient, but I pray he was pain free.

Morphine has received a bad reputation as the "death drug", but it is not unless misused. I am often asked if we use morphine as a form of euthanasia, but it is not my choice or a doctor's choice to hasten death. I believe death is God's choice. Hospice physicians for severe pain prescribe morphine. It has been my experience with every patient that morphine is started at a low dose and adjusted as needed. Morphine is a unique drug that works wonders if taken as prescribed (carenotkilling.org.uk).

Difficulty Breathing

Everyone knows what air is: It is in the atmosphere and always around us. It's something we don't think about until we are without it. When patients have difficulty breathing, it causes anxiety for the family. Unfortunately, many patients become short of breath. Even patients with no lung problems may develop shortness of breath.

As soon as a patient developed shortness of breath, I would call our hospice physician to get an order for oxygen and antianxiety medication.

These are a few things I used to help patients with shortness of breath:

- It is very important to keep the patient calm. Increased anxiety increases shortness of breath.
- The head of the bed should be raised.
- Place a fan blowing directly on the patient, as tolerated.
- The room should be cool, as cool as can be tolerated.
- Place a moist cloth on the forehead.
- Pain should be controlled. The more pain, the harder it is to breath.
- The atmosphere should be quiet and relaxing. Play soft music from the patient's younger years, and dim the lights.
- Don't leave the patient alone; with increased shortness of breath comes increased fear and anxiety.

- Don't force food or liquids. Offer non-greasy food and sips of water.

When a patient starts to make the transition to actively dying, the patient may develop shallow breathing with a collection of fluid in the lungs. This may make a rattling sound and is called the "death rattle." It is a natural process and is expected, but not all patients develop the death rattle.

As scary is witnessing this is for caregivers, experiencing shortness of breath is even more terrifying for the patient. When my daughter was six months and my son was five years old, I was in a fabric store. I was going to dash in and dash out, so there was no need to bother with a stroller. I walked in carrying my daughter in my arms, and my son walked by my side. I quickly looked through the aisles, and when I got to the back of the store, I started coughing and could not catch my breath. I was not choking, but there was something microscopic in my lungs and my body was fiercely trying to get it out. I struggled to get air back in my lungs. My eyes poured water in some type of allergic fit. I sat my daughter on a table of remnant fabrics and I coughed while watching my son run around the store, but I could do nothing. I felt totally helpless as I stood there, unable to breathe. If someone had snatched my son, I would not have been able to save him. I coughed non-stop for what seemed like an hour, but I'm sure it was only a few minutes. With every cough, I gasped for air. People looked at me as if I had a disease, and not one person offered to help. Even with a baby and a five-year-old, no one offered to help. I was mortified with the lack of caring from my fellow Americans.

Finally, a lady asked if I would like a mint. I nodded my head, still coughing and gasping. The mint was a miracle. I stopped coughing, picked up my daughter and son, and left the store as quickly as I could. I drove straight home. I was exhausted. The energy it took to cough and try to breathe was astronomical.

I was healthy and, thank God, I had no health issues. I don't know why I had the breathing episode that day, but every time I'm with a patient who can't breathe, I remember that terrible day. I have often wondered if God allowed me to have this scary experience so

I would have a tiny idea of what my patients go through when they can't breathe. When I shared my experience with Chaplain Ron, he agreed that God had a purpose for that episode.

Other Common Symptoms

<u>Nausea and Vomiting</u>
Hospice physicians can prescribe medications to control nausea and vomiting.

<u>Constipation</u>
Medications, lack of physical activity, and decreased fluid intake can cause constipation. Increase fluid intake. Offer water and apple juice. Avoid cheese and peanut butter. If constipation continues, report the symptom to the nurse, and hospice physicians may prescribe a stool softener or laxative.

<u>Diarrhea</u>
Loose stools and abdominal cramping is not pleasant. If diarrhea lasts more than two hours, the patient may become dehydrated. It is important not to consume caffeine. Decrease the intake of fruit, vegetables, and dairy products. If diarrhea continues after making changes to the diet, the patient may need a prescription to stop the diarrhea.

Home

Written by Michelle

Many people believe hospice patients spend their last days in a Hospice House or hospital. Hospice patients may live with family or friends, live in a nursing facility, or go to a Hospice House. They may live at home and can live anywhere they call home. You may be surprised where many people call home and what their home environment is like.

During my career, I have been to many homes. I had patients that lived in beautiful ocean front condominiums, beautiful lake homes, plantation homes on hundreds of acres, little homes, sweet homes, average homes, run down homes, hotels, run-down apartments, unsanitary homes, and even cars. However, each one has housed someone who needed me and deserved a painless exit to heaven.

I had a patient that lived in an old, small, home in the rough part of town. The home was clean, but had an old smell. When I walked into the home for the first time, I noticed the old curtains. The print was a flower and through the years the color had faded in the sun to a dingy light beige. As I looked around, the furniture looked at least one hundred years old, and they were not fine antiques by any means.

He was ninety years old and had heart and lung problems. I had many weekly visits with this patient and I enjoyed his company. He was smart, lonely, and very poor. I learned he married around the age of twenty, his wife cheated around the age of twenty-one, and he divorced at twenty-two. I learned he never remarried because he stayed home and took care of his parents until they died. By the time his parents were in heaven, he was too old to remarry and had health problems. If you are around a patient long enough, you end up talking about yourself, too, and I told him I loved potato chips; they were my favorite snack, and I would choose them over chocolate any day. The next week I arrived at his home, and he had a small, single-portion bag of potato chips. Hospice employees are not supposed to accept gifts and money from our patients, but it was common to receive a cake, pie, or cookies. At Christmas, I always received small gifts such as gift towels, hand sanitizers, scented lotions and soaps from patients. I would accept small gifts, but never money. I loved that the patients thought enough of me to give me a token of appreciation, and those potato chips meant the world to me. That small bag of potato chips was my favorite gift I ever received from a patient because he barely had the money to buy food for himself, but he thought of me.

Another home was small and old, but clean and critter and clutter free. During my first visit, I was directed to the kitchen where the patient was having lunch. All was normal until I walked into the kitchen where, to my surprise, there was a huge crack in the floor. The crack ran from one side to the other, and was approximately a foot wide. The patient was sitting at the table on the side of the crack closest to the front door. The patient used a walker and had problems ambulating. In order to go to the other side of the kitchen, you would have to jump over the crack in the floor.

I asked, "How does your mother get to the other side of the kitchen and the rest of the house?"

The patient's daughter stated, "She doesn't go on that side of the house". She explained that the house had settled years ago and they did not have the money to fix the crack. In my opinion, the house should have been condemned, but it was not my job to inspect the house. I was there to ensure the patient was safe and getting the appropriate care. The patient was well cared for and had all she needed on one side of the house. She did not have to cross the crack, so I let it go and said a thank you to God for giving me a home without any major cracks in the floor.

I actually visited many run-down homes with holes in the floor. One home was very old, but when I walked in the front door, the home was spotless and smelled clean. I could smell bleach, and nothing was out of place. The patient was on the couch and, as I walked toward her, I noticed a foot-wide hole in the floor. I thought, how odd. I would have put a rug over the hole or possibly a piece of furniture, but there it was: a hole in the middle of the room. I wanted to ask about the hole, but the family acted as if there was no hole and the patient had no bruises, so I said nothing. The patient was cared for and the house was clean, so I did not ask about the hole.

I have worked in bug-infested homes—many bug-infested homes. I could write a whole book on bugs. During my assessments, I had to check the patient's medications. In one home, I was given the patient's medications in a plastic bag. When I opened the bag, there were five dead bugs in the bag. I thanked God the bugs were dead, because I probably would have had a heart attack if the bugs had been alive and had crawled on my hand.

There were many dog and cat infested homes. One apartment had approximately fifty cats and during one visit a cat jumped on the kitchen table and urinated in a bowl of fruit. I pretended I did not witness that action. Some things are better left alone.

I had a patient who had a five-foot alligator as a pet. The patient lived in the country and the alligator lived in the concrete pool in his backyard. The pool had a fence and the alligator could not get out. The alligator had an amazing life and was fed the finest cuts of meat. He was fat and happy.

My fondest memory took place with a patient that lived in a nursing home. My patient had dementia and many other health problems. She was approximately 6 foot tall and stayed to herself barely talking to anyone. You could see her all day, every day, in her wheel chair. She would slowly propel herself down the long hallways. The facility had many activities for their patients, but she didn't want anything to do with anyone and refused to participate in the activities. One day I found her in the dining room. Her wheelchair was parked in front of the television and she was singing with Elvis Presley. Presley was in concert and singing *"How Great Thou Art"*.

This lady couldn't tell you what her name was, but she was singing every word of the song. She sang out loud and raised her hands up to God to the lyrics, *"oh Lord my God"*. She would place her hands to her ears as she sang the lyrics, *"I hear the rolling thunder"*. Place her hands on her chest as she sang, 'then sings my soul". As the song ended with "how great thou art", she placed her face in her hands and wept. It was beautiful and I cried as I watched her. I was in shock and amazed. I knew very little about this patient because she had no living relatives and she was confused. Before that day, I only had clinical information on this patient. After that day, I knew everything I needed to know, I knew where her soul was going.

I had a patient who lived in a run-down hotel that had been converted into apartments. It was a dump and crack dealers sold drugs on each side of the converted apartment. After my first visit, I was not happy. I went to my supervisor and said, "We should not be admitting patients who live in converted, run-down apartments with drug dealers on each corner."

She looked me dead in the eye and said, "Maybe this is not the right place for you to work. Look at all your patients. Which one needs you the most?"

I lowered my head and walked out of her office because she was correct. That patient needed me and our hospice services more than any of my other patients at that time. I was embarrassed and ashamed because I had been selfish. The patient was a recovered addict, she was forty years old, but looked sixty. She was diagnosed with lung cancer, had no family, and all her friends were the drug dealers on the corner. Not one drug dealer said one word to me. Not one of her neighbors bothered me or caused me harm. I believe they knew I was there to help their neighbor and friend. During my visits, I never felt completely safe, but I never felt afraid. This patient needed our hospice team and we provided the best care possible and she did not die alone. She died pain free with dignity and respect.

I had a patient who lived in the projects, and one night she called when I was on-call. It was no fun driving to the bad side of town in the middle of the night, but she was having trouble breathing. She lived alone, and she was afraid of dying. When

I arrived, the neighbors were all awake and very interested. The elderly patient with lung disease was having trouble breathing and had tremendous anxiety. After a breathing treatment, she was breathing better and I left. I was nervous walking to my car. It was late and I walked quickly. My car was in one piece, but the car's emblem was stolen from the front of my car. I could not believe someone had the nerve to steal my car's emblem. I believe it was a teenager being silly because if someone wanted to steal something, they would have broken into my car. The emblem cost approximately fifty dollars to replace. It cost me more to work that night than if I had not worked.

For the most part, I have found people have respect for hospice and those of us who chose to work in the business of caring for others.

Homeless to Home

Let not your heart be troubled: ye believe in God, believe also in me.
In my Father's house are many mansions: if it were not so, I would have told you. I go to prepare a place for you.
And if I go and prepare a place for you, I will come again, and receive you unto myself; that where I am, there ye may be also.
— **John 14:1-3**

Written by Michelle

I was sitting in my usual seat for the Monday morning meeting and the nurse who was on-call for the weekend gave a report on a patient she had admitted.

I was busy catching up on my charting from the previous week, so I was listening with one ear. The nurse was unsettled about a patient she had admitted over the weekend. He was homeless, living in his van, and had face cancer. He had a tumor on the side of his face that was open and draining. Of course, there was no running water, and the condition of the van was unsanitary to say the least. Wound care needed to be performed twice per day and in America wound care should be done with clean hands—not necessarily sterile conditions, but clean to prevent further problems with infection. At that point, infection was our primary concern.

Our social workers were hard at work trying to get the patient placed in a nursing facility.

I knew his case was bad, but I was a seasoned nurse that had always asked for the wound care cases everywhere I had worked. Nothing shocked me and nothing bothered me in the way of wounds. The social worker finally got the patient placed in a skilled nursing facility and I was assigned to his case because he was now in my territory.

I was eager to meet the patient and take a look at the wound I had heard so much about. I walked into the room and was in shock. I could not believe what I was looking at. The sight was like something out of a horror show. I should not have been shocked, I had seen thousands of wounds in the past and heard many reports on this patient for months. I don't know how the patient survived two months in his state, and in an unclean environment, but thank God, he was moved to a facility with a bed, running water, and nursing care. His wounds were cleaned and dressed three times per day, and he was given pain medication when he was in pain. It was a blessing for me to see this man receiving the care and respect he deserved while on this earth.

Written by Chaplain Ron

After hearing what Michelle told me about this case, I didn't know what to expect when I entered the nursing home to visit the patient. From the description of his sores and wounds described by Michelle and other team members, I prayed to God for strength. I had heard that he was homeless prior to his placement in the facility and knew that he was suffering. When I entered into his room, he was lying there and acknowledged my presence. And although his face was deteriorating as Michelle and the other team members had described, as I looked him in his eyes I thanked God for allowing me to see beyond the physical man, for what I saw was a dying man. I reached out my hand, and asked if he was a believer in God, and he said yes. I affirmed his faith and salvation through Jesus Christ and we recited the "Our Father" prayer together:

Our Father who art in heaven, hollowed will be thy name, thy kingdom come thy will be done, on earth as it is in heaven, give us this day our daily bread and forgive us our trespasses as we forgive who trespass against us, and lead us not into temptation, but deliver us from evil, for thine is the kingdom, and the power, and the glory, forever, Amen……

A few days later, the patient passed. I then realized that although he went from being homeless and living in a van, to being moved to a facility, both places were only his temporary homes. and would again be homeless here on earth. For as I witnessed him cry out, "*Abba Father*," Jesus Christ had prepared for him a permanent home, an eternal resting place, a place where there would be no more tears, pain, suffering nor sorrow, because this place was his mansion in heaven.

Words For Thought From Chaplain Ron

Although it may be difficult to imagine and anticipate how our homes will be like without our presence or the presence of a loved one when that appointed time shall come, a time that we all must face in our lives, remember the words of Jesus Christ and the promise that He has made unto us. *Let not your heart be troubled*. For all who believe in Him, he is preparing for us an everlasting mansion in heaven as we all too one day, will be home-less here on earth.

Forgiven

Verily I say unto you, All sins shall be forgiven unto the sons of men, and blasphemies wherewith soever they shall blaspheme:
But he that shall blaspheme against the Holy Ghost hath never forgiveness, but is in danger of eternal damnation.
—Mark 3:28-29

Written by Michelle

I had a cardiopulmonary patient who also suffered from Post-Traumatic Stress Disorder or PTSD (*merriam-webster.com*). He told me he served in the trenches and had killed many men. The words PTSD never came out of his mouth and I don't believe he understood what PTSD was. I believe he felt God was punishing him.

He told me about his terrifying and reoccurring dream. The dream would start out in a beautiful pool. He and his family were enjoying the time in the sun and were playing games in the pool. The dream would turn from the pool to a lake. Many boats would go back and forth. The lake was full of people swimming and skiing. Suddenly, the beautiful blue water would turn to a nasty murk. He would be in the lake swimming and a dead body would appear. The body always had long, red hair, and he never saw the face. His body would get caught in the hair and he could not get loose. The hair would drag him down into the water, and he would start drowning. He would wake up in a sweaty panic.

He told a story about fighting an enemy soldier and how he fought for his life. He tried to strangle the enemy, but he wasn't at war, he was in his bed and was strangling his wife. The only way she survived was by picking up the telephone and hitting him on the head. When he woke, he had to deal with the tragedy that he had almost killed his wife. He said his life was never the same after that night. He was never able to sleep in the same bed with his wife and his secret was now out in the open. He hid his dreams and his horror from his family for many years. He felt it was a sign of weakness, and many years ago PTSD was unheard of.

During one of my visits, we talked about God. He looked me square in the eye and asked for my opinion on killing during war. I was very uncomfortable, because I'm not a biblical scholar. I will talk all day about how good God has been to me, but I'm not going to preach on a subject I know nothing about. I explained I did not know enough about biblical war, but I stated that God killed during biblical times. I remembered a sermon I once heard about not having to fight our battles because God would fight our battles for us. In this story, God fought and killed the enemy.

His eyes did not budge, and he was waiting for my opinion. My heart broke into a million pieces. I could see and feel his pain. His guilt was enormous. I grabbed his hands and squeezed them because I wanted to be sure he was listening to me. I explained that it did not matter what he had done in the past. "God is a forgiving God," I explained. "God would forgive murder and any other sin you have committed." As I squeezed his hands, I prayed out loud. I prayed that God would grant him peace and mercy.

Unfortunately, I did not remember the chapter and verses that day, but Chaplain Ron showed me where to find it:

"And when they began to sing and praise, the Lord set an ambush against the men of Ammon, Moab, and Mount Seir, who had come against Judah, so that they were routed" (2 Chronicles 20:22).

PTSD is a real disorder that occurs after experiencing a shocking, dangerous, or traumatic event. It can develop after serving in a war or any traumatizing episode. When we are in difficult situations, our bodies produce chemicals to help us fight or run. It is called fight or flight and is a mechanism to help our bodies defend themselves. Most people recover from traumatic events, but many don't. It is individualized and someone may have a mild traumatic event and not recover, while another person may experience a major traumatic event and have no future problems from the event. Many people relive the event or suffer other symptoms such as nightmares, depression, or guilt for many years, and some till the day they die. Many veterans suffer from PTSD because they fought many life-or-death battles.

Words for thought from Chaplain Ron

Be encouraged not to let what you have done in the past take away the joy and happiness that the Lord is offering you today. For Jesus said in the third chapter of Mark that there is only one unpardonable sin. God is faithful and just, and is willing to forgive all who come to Him with a repenting heart.

Timesharing

Live joyfully with the wife whom thou lovest all the days of the life of thy vanity which he hath give thee under the sun.
—**Ecclesiastes 9:9a**

Written by Chaplain Ron

At this point in our careers, Michelle was the clinical director of our hospice office. I remember her getting a call from another office four hours away. The office requested a temporary transfer of an Alzheimer's patient because her husband wanted to bring her to their timeshare in Myrtle Beach. This was odd because the patient was in the late stages of the disease. Michelle was not happy and tried to stop the transfer. She felt the trip would be too stressful for the patient, and she was worried the patient may not survive the long drive. The husband, however, insisted. Michelle was overruled and the husband and the patient made several trips back and forth over three months. While the patient was in Myrtle Beach, we were responsible for overseeing the patient's care.

One day I received a call from Michelle that the patient had passed, and I needed to go to their timeshare immediately. When I arrived, the husband was packing their personal belongings and shared with me how his wife loved the beach. Of all the places they had vacationed over the years, this was her favorite. With tears in his eyes, he looked at me and said, "This timeshare is the best investment I ever made for our family. We've spent time with our children traveling to many places. We have so many memories enjoying one another. The reason I brought her back-and-forth from here-to-there, is because this is where she wanted to spend her last days. Although I didn't know when that time would come, all I could do was put it in God's hands. What she desired, He has honored, and I thank God for the blessing of this timeshare."

Words for Thought from Chaplain Ron

The time that we have to share with our loved ones is a blessing and is more precious than anything we could ever imagine. Be encouraged to use this time wisely in creating loving memories that will be with us for the rest of our lives and generations to come.

Alzheimer's

Happy is the man that findeth wisdom, and the man that getteth understanding.
—**Proverbs 3: 13**

Written by Michelle

According to the Alzheimer's Association, more than five million Americans are living with Alzheimer's. By 2050, this number could rise as high as sixteen million *(www.alz.org/facts/overview.asp)*.

Alzheimer's disease is a silent killer. Because the disease process can take years, seeing patients and their families go through this experience can be challenging.

Till Death Do Us Part

During my career, I had two cases where a husband and wife died within a short period of time of each other.

In the first case, the husband had been paralyzed for many years and had many pressure wounds, often referred to as bed sores. Pressure wounds are very common in elderly, paralyzed patients. This couple had a wonderful family who took care of them around the clock. I assessed the two patients and admitted them to our hospice. Both were in bad shape, and although the husband had many wounds, I felt the wife would die first because she had more health problems. One night I was on-call and received a call at 11:00 pm. The family reported the husband was in severe pain. Before this night, the patient did not have severe pain. The sudden increase in pain was not a good sign. The family stated they had administered all the appropriate pain medications. I called my wonderful hospice physician and he asked me to go by his home to pick up a prescription for morphine. I picked up the prescription and had it filled at a twenty-four-hour pharmacy. I delivered and administered the medication. The patient's pain was relieved and he was blessed to die pain-free. His wife was confused, but in an unusual fate, she died a month later. I have often said that I believe she and her husband were so in love that they could not live without each other. Even though the wife was confused and in the late stages of Alzheimer's, I believe she knew her husband was not on this earth.

In the second case, the husband had late stage Alzheimer's disease. His wife was elderly and physically disabled, but she was not ill. She was surprisingly healthy and only the husband was admitted to our hospice. During my visits, I met many family members, friends, and a ton of church friends. This man was loved in his community and everyone knew him. As time went by, the patient grew weaker and weaker. On the day he went to heaven, his wife assured me she would be fine. She had much support and loved everyone. She adored her children, grand-children, and great-grandchildren. She had so much to live for, but she had a broken heart. Two months later, I received a call from her daughter and was told her mother had died. I was in shock. The daughter explained that her mother did not feel well and was taken to the local emergency room. The doctors started running test and she was diagnosed with cancer. The daughter stated there was no time to call for hospice or anyone else. Her mother died a day later. Her daughter stated, "She died of a broken heart." I believe the daughter was correct.

I had a friend whose parents were diagnosed with Alzheimer's Disease and dementia, and they died three weeks apart. I asked about his experience:

> "Death is a subject that we think about throughout our lives, but often its impact does not affect us directly. The deaths we witness are in the movies, on a news report of a car accident, or in a warzone. It

always happens, it seems, to someone else's family. Your own life clock seems to keep ticking just fine. Even when you eventually lose a grandparent the phrase, "it was their time to go," sounds like it was an event prepackaged and arranged long before you came along. The connection between their time and your time is not a conversation anyone has at the funeral when you are a grandchild. It's a cushiony time/mind barrier from our own mortal soul. But when you lose *both* of your own parents, you are not fully in the equation. Your very essence seems to lose all foundation. At that same moment, your own life clock begins ticking. You knew you had a life clock around somewhere, but it never ticked this loudly. Your buffer from the end of days has been dropped. You have been tagged. You have just lost life- long loves who shared all the good, great, and bad things you have been through. Losing both parents eliminates your best and most caring support system. On top of that, God just handed you the family stopwatch.

"I thought I was prepared for the eventual death of my mother and dad. My mom had had non-Hodgkin's lymphoma twice and still survived for seventeen years. My dad had had a quadruple bypass and numerous stents over twenty years. So, I knew they could possibly pass at any time, right? After these ailments, they went the usual route of being in an assisted living center and then a nursing home. Then my mother developed Alzheimer's and my dad dementia. So, for three or four of their final years our telephone calls or conversations of substance became nil. But even after all of this, I was still never prepared for this call from my brother. "You will probably take this harder than anyone.....Dad died today." Then just three weeks later, I received the same call about Mom.

"Sure, everyone has the patented clichés we all have heard. 'We are so sorry for your loss.' 'They are in a better place.' 'They are now with the angels.' 'They are watching over you tonight.' Well, those are all nice comforting statements, but for the time being I was more interested in real biology. What happened? How does a body die? What were they thinking as they died? What were they feeling? Does God have a natural morphine for the brain to take them to their eternal rest? Is that why they say your life flashes before your eyes? Was there a lot pain? Were they scared? Did they know they were dying? Is the brain really the last thing to go? Did they have a few minutes or hours where they rallied? Did they say anything of value as they parted? I didn't want a family member to color these moments for me with their bias. I wanted real answers about these things from medical personnel, a hospice nurse or doctor or someone who had witnessed many of these final moments of life before. Was the way in which my mother and dad died normal? Is there such a thing as normal? Did every professional who had witnessed death before know exactly what was happening to my parents as they died? Those are questions we don't discuss nearly enough. I wonder, why?

"I will have the rest of my life to figure out what it all means. I will spend hours driving in my car thinking about them. I'll spend years, hopefully, talking to friends and loved ones and family members. Together we can attempt to sort out what their lives and deaths meant to those they touched or brought into this world.

"Unfortunately, no one will ever understand the real me as well as my parents. No one, even in matrimony, may be able to fully exalt as much in my successes or hurt, as much along with me in my tribulations. My love for them and all they did to raise me was never underappreciated. So at least I have comfort that I was always a good son. I have those thoughts to keep me warm. But the newness of steering my own ship without the usual rudders is still strange and lonely. And this final destination timeline, that I used to ignore, has now magnified the importance and turn of every sail."

The Great Escape

Written by Michelle

While I worked for a hospice company, we had a demented patient to get out of a home in the middle of July. In South Carolina, the temperatures in July can get to 100 degrees and, at times, the heat index can reach 130 degrees. The elderly patient lived with his daughter on a farm. Acres of woods and farmland surrounded the home. Everyone knew this patient would not live long in the sweltering heat. The patient was not my patient, but I received a call to go to the area immediately. Everyone was joining the search. When I arrived, there were police and firemen everywhere and a search-and-rescue was under way. The patient's family, friends, and church members were also searching. We were sent home because there was more than enough help. Two hours later, the patient was found in a cornfield down a dirt road not far from his home. He was taken to the hospital and received IV fluids and safely returned home in a few days.

During my hospice career, I only had one of my patients escape. The patient was an elderly lady with Alzheimer's disease. I arrived at the patient's home on a hot afternoon in June. The patient's husband was standing outside their oceanfront condominium. He was disabled and could barely walk, so he was standing out front asking neighbors to look for his wife. He was very upset because it was hot, she could get on the street and get hit by a car, could meet someone who would potentially could harm her, or could get in the ocean and drown. He was very upset and barely could talk due to crying. My training was in nursing, not search-and-rescue, but I flipped a switch and turned into Superwoman.

In my scrubs and nursing shoes, I dashed out to the highway and recruited help. There were many people walking around. Some were walking their dogs, others were walking along the sidewalk to a local pub. Many people were in the parking lot loading and unloading luggage.

Everyone was running up and down the road, recruiting others to help in the search as well. My main concern was to make sure the patient did not get hit by a car if she was on the street. Once the street was covered with my recruits, I dashed over to the beach. I ran up and down the beach like a mad woman. My nursing shoes were full of sand, and everyone on the beach looked at me like I was a demented person, running up and down the beach in my full nursing uniform. It wasn't long until I had recruits searching on the beach. We quickly had searchers going to the right and searchers going to left of the beach.

There were several sets of grey condominiums that were identical to the patient's condominium, so I started a search party in those condos as well. I found the patient a few doors down at another condominium complex. Thank God, she was safe and we had a good outcome.

Unfortunately, there are times it is difficult to contain a confused person. This patient was a huge safety risk and the escape opened the husband's eyes and he placed the patient in a nursing home the next week. His heart was broken and he was devastated, but it was the right thing to do for her safety.

Words For Thought From Chaplain Ron

There may come a time as caregivers where we are not able to provide the necessary level of care for our loved ones. Choices and decisions that must be made at this time require prayer and education. Although this may be the most difficult decision ever made during your time together, it a blessing to be able to have your loved on in a safe and secure environment.

I Still Remember

Then I said, I will not make mention of him, nor speak any more in his name. But his word was in my heart as a burning fire shut up in my bones.
—Jeremiah 20:9a

Written by Chaplain Ron

At the point in the disease process that individuals meet criteria for hospice care, they have lost the ability to hold a meaningful conversation and are only able to speak a couple of words. I remember visiting a patient who was a very devout church-goer and Christian woman. During my visits with her, she would be lying in bed, sometimes with her eyes open, other times not, and would only mumble something that I could not understand from time to time. I would sit by her bedside and sing hymns, read Scripture, and pray the "Our Father" prayer out loud before departing. One day during my visit when I was reciting the prayer, I got to the end and she uttered, "On earth." Although I had finished the prayer when she said this, it brought great joy to my heart just to hear her say those two words of the prayer. This was surely God's confirmation that although this disease destroys one's cognitive abilities over time, what she had learned many years ago as the model prayer unto our Father who art in heaven is hidden deep down in her heart, mind, and soul, and will never be forgotten.

Words for thought from Chaplain Ron

Individuals with Alzheimer's disease still maintain some long-term memory. When providing spiritual care, sing hymns for comfort that are very old in order to spiritually connect with them. Also, although there are many new translations of the Bible for better understanding, always read from the KJV. Saying the "Our Father" prayer will also help to trigger spiritual and religious activities of the past.

Go Tigers!

Delight thyself also in the Lord; and he shall give thee the desires of thine heart.
                                              —*Psalm 37:4*

Written by Chaplain Ron

I am a big sports fan and from time to time throughout my career, I would meet patients who shared in the same love of sports. My son was a Division 1 football recruit out of high school and during his recruiting years I had the opportunity to meet many college coaches and recruiters. During my son's college football career, I thank God for the opportunity that I had to be a road chaplain and deliver the devotion messages following the team's dinner the night before the games.

I'll never forget being assigned a patient who was diagnosed with prostate cancer, and when I made my first visit the first thing that I noticed was that his house was decorated with pennants and pictures of his favorite college football team. He was a huge fan, and after we talked about God we always had another conversation about football. During every visit month after month we would recap a game or play "Monday morning quarterback." I looked forward to my visits with him, and the excitement in his voice when we talked about his team, let me know that he enjoyed it too.

After several months, as his disease began to progress, he became weaker and was not able to hold lengthy conversations. One day when I made my visit, he could barely mumble a few words. It was not easy to look at my friend who I enjoyed talking sports with not be able to hold a conversation with me anymore, but I thank God for the times that he could. As I sat by his bedside that day, his wife came over to me and said, "Do you know what he has asked for?"

I replied, "No, but please tell me."

"He would like an autographed photo of the Tigers coach".

"Really?" I said. "Let me see what I can do." It was not a coincidence but God's blessing that the coach was someone that I had personally met and spent a lot of time with because he had been actively trying to recruit my son. When I got back to the office, I called his office and asked his secretary if she could give him a message that I needed an autographed photo of him sent to the home of my patient who only had a short time to live.

The next day I got a call from my patient's wife who was so excited that a Fed-Ex package had arrived and the photo was there. I rushed over and was filled with joy to see it hanging on the wall over his bed as God had blessed him with one of his heart's last desires.

And from that time on, every time college football season comes around, I can't help but think about him. And last year, when his team won the national championship, I could only imagine what a joyful conversation we would have had if he had still been living. But deep down in my heart, I believe that although he had traveled many times over the years to watch his favorite team play in the stadium called "Death Valley," he was watching that championship game from the grandstand seats of heaven. And on that final play, when the game had been won in the final seconds, he was looking down from heaven, and saying, *"Go Tigers!"*

Grief

Then saith he unto them, My soul is exceeding sorrowful, even unto death: tarry ye here, and watch with me.
And he went a little farther, and fell on his face, and prayed, saying, O my Father, if it be possible, let this cup pass from me: nevertheless not as I will, but as thou wilt.
He went away again the second time, and prayed, saying, O my Father, if this cup may not pass away from me, except I drink it, thy will be done.

—**Matthew 26:38-39, 42**

Written by Michelle

Time, they say, heals all wounds. How long and how much time? That is the million-dollar question, and there is no magic number. The time depends on the individual circumstance. I can say from experience, there are many factors to healing and many types of grief. The grief I witnessed was normal grief, anticipatory grief, and chronic grief.

Normal grief is a gift from God. In my opinion, grief allows us to mourn a loss then move forward to a new life. Normal grieving consists of sadness and acceptance—acceptance of the death and a new life. After a loss, nothing will be the same, but the new life can be good.

Anticipatory grief is grief before a person dies. I have witnessed anticipatory grief from patients and caregivers. It is very easy for a terminally ill patient and caregiver to say, "I wish I had done this", or "I wish I had not done that". It is normal and expected to be sad about a terminal diagnosis, but death of life should not occur before a person dies.

I had a patient diagnosed with heart disease. He lived in a tiny house outside of town. It was the smallest home I had ever been to. His home had one bedroom, one bathroom, a tiny kitchen with a couch and television. He and his wife lived together and were very much in love. He adored his wife, and he loved his life. He did not want to die. With every visit, he grew weaker. With every visit, his worrying grew stronger.

He was a man of God and always had a large, black, worn Bible at his side. His Bible was falling apart. He told of how many times he had read the Bible cover to cover and of how he had previously volunteered in his church. Now his sick body was unable to attend church. He and his wife did not have much, but they were happy with what little they had. He did not want material things; he wanted a life with his wife. His wife was also sick, but worked to help make ends meet. The patient was not physically able to hold down a job, but he tried to clean the house or would at the least try to do laundry. All he wanted to do was to help his wife. His body was very weak and he could barely walk from the bedroom to the kitchen.

Every visit was full of crying. He cried and cried. He worried and worried. He grieved and grieved. He worried about dying and leaving his wife with nothing. He worried about living and not being able to help his wife. She was a lovely woman and all she wanted was for him to have peace. During every visit, we discussed faith and the power of God. He always stated he had faith in God, but he was full of anxiety and full of grief. After every visit, I was mentally exhausted. His fear and anxiety would rub off on me. I feel I am a positive person, but I know from personal experience that negativity is very powerful. Satan uses negative thoughts to bring doubt and to cause a lack of faith. I believe Satan used negativity to tear this man down. Every visit with this patient was exhausting, but I loved this patient. He was grieving his death to the point that he could not live. None of us know how many days we have on this earth, so it's important to try and enjoy life. I so badly wanted to see this patient live his last days with a smile and not tears, but that is something I did not get to see. This patient did not spend his last days living, he lived his last days dying.

Chronic grieving is grieving that doesn't end. It usually leads to hopelessness and depression. Usually the chronic griever grieves over what they feel they could have done while the patient was alive. Many times, they grieve over what they feel they could have done to help the patient to live longer. There have been times a caregiver mourns the death of a loved one and forgets that the doctors, nurses, and even he himself do not hold the power of life. Only God holds that power.

I once had a patient who was diagnosed with liver failure. He had taken a prescription for high cholesterol that damaged his liver. I arrived at his mobile home for the first time to complete his admission, and his son started screaming at me, "You people have killed my father!" I was in shock because no one had ever talked to me that way in a professional setting. I had not prescribed the medication; I had not administered the medication. I was there to help his dying father. I was not there to perform a screaming match or to try to figure out what caused the damage to his father's liver. The son's mother walked him to another room, and I completed my assessment. Unfortunately, the patient had severe liver damage and would not live long. The son was not able to work due to his grief and stayed with his dad night and day. He had many fits of anger. During every visit, he screamed and would throw household items around the room. He was angry at me, angry at God, but most of all he was angry at himself for allowing his dad to take the medication that caused his condition. I respectfully say that this son had no medical training and there was no way he could have recommended his dad not take the medication. I never saw the son after his father's death, but the bereavement coordinator stayed in touch to try to help this man with his chronic grief.

God is a loving and forgiving God. Whatever was or was not done should not be allowed to ruin a future. God allows us to grieve for a reason and I believe it is to bring us closer to Him. I believe grief is intended to bring us to a point that we see that God is in control.

I remember studying grief many years ago in nursing school. The model my school used was Dr. Kubler-Ross's Five Stages of Grief, but there are many other models from other doctors. Many use Dr. Kubler-Ross's basic five stages of grief, but they add stages to better explain the grieving process. I have witnessed all stages in my career and personal life.

Dr. Kubler-Ross's five stages of grief:

1. Denial - Unable to accept the news that there is a diagnosis of a terminal illness. The person may believe the news is not true and everything will soon return to normal. The person may be in shock and unable to think clearly.
2. Anger - Once reality sets in, the realization that the illness is terminal usually brings anger that this could happen to them or to their loved one. The person may carry the weight of the world on their shoulders.
3. Bargaining - People usually ask God to change the diagnosis. They try to bargain with God stating they will change certain behaviors and life choices if God will make them or their loved one well.
4. Depression - When it's evident that denial, anger, and bargaining are not going to change the diagnosis, people may become depressed and become helpless. During this stage, a world of emotions occurs. There may be crying, changes in sleep, refusing to attend social gatherings, refusing to accept visitors, and changes in appetite.
5. Acceptance - The time usually comes when the individual is ready to move forward and make a plan for the end and will usually be ready to get their affairs in order *(Psychcentral.com)*.

Each stage is individual and takes different amounts of time for each person to accomplish.

We Grieve In Different Ways

Written by Michelle

I had a patient who was diagnosed with breast cancer. The patient was admitted to hospice and was given a few weeks to live. The youngest daughter lived next door and was best friends with her mother. They did everything together. Once the patient was diagnosed, the daughter would not visit or communicate with her mother. The other children were outraged and could not understand how the youngest sibling could be heartless and uncaring.

We grieve in different ways. The youngest daughter was heartbroken and withdrew into her own world. She did not visit her mother for two weeks and when her mother died, she had no interest in the funeral arrangements. She had nothing to be guilty for, she was a wonderful daughter, but she could not handle being a part of her mother's last days. She attended the funeral and was beyond devastated. She loved her mother, and she grieved the way she had to grieve.

There are times we need to step back and not judge, but understand that we all grieve in different ways. What is important is that a person moves forward, stage-by-stage, and makes it to the fifth stage and accepts.

Words For Thought From Chaplain Ron

During his life on earth and journey to the cross, Jesus as a physical man like you and I, in the shortest verse in the bible found in the 11th chapter of John, shed tears over Jerusalem. In Matthew chapter 26, he expressed his sorrow regarding death to his disciples, and in his initial prayer in the garden, pleaded to God to take the cup of suffering and death away from him. As he prayed a second time, he overcame his anticipatory grief and accepted his Father's will. It is okay to shed tears, be afraid of death, or be upset at losing a loved one. Be encouraged to seek spiritual strength, for he knows all about it and will be with you along your journey. Remember the grieving words of David in Psalm 23, verse 4: *"Ye though I walk through the valley of the shadow of death, I will fear no evil: for thou art with me, thy rod and thy staff they comfort me."*

A Change of Mind

For God so loved the world, that he gave his only begotten Son, that whosoever believeth in him should not perish, but have everlasting life.

– John.3:16

Written by Michelle

Medicare requires that a hospice agency employs a physician, nurse, chaplain, and social worker. When I started working with hospice, I thought requiring a chaplain was a waste of taxpayers' dollars. Some patients decline the chaplain services. They may have their own pastor, or not want to hear about religion.

In 2009, I had a patient who was diagnosed with late-stage prostate cancer. He declined chaplain services and was not interested in God or religion. With every visit, I asked the patient if he would like a visit from the chaplain. I explained that the chaplain was a wonderful person who talked about everything from religion to sports and would enjoy listening to any problems he may have. Essentially, I explained the chaplain could be a friend. Finally, he agreed to one visit. Only one visit.

After Chaplain Ron visited the patient, he wanted more visits and the chaplain visited his home twice per month for several months.

The family was blessed with one last Thanksgiving. I was on-call and received a call the day after Thanksgiving that the patient was declining rapidly. After assessing the patient, the near-death signs were present. The family asked to see Chaplain Ron. I called Chaplain Ron and he was on his way back from Maryland.

The Last Blessing

He had been visiting with family for Thanksgiving. He dropped his wife and children off at their home, and he drove straight to the patient's home.

The family was very concerned about where their father's soul would go. Chaplain Ron explained to the family that their father had a change of mind during an earlier visit. There was no doubt that their loved one would soon be in heaven. He explained how he had held his hand as he listened to God's simple plan for salvation and accepted Jesus Christ as his Lord and Savior.

I witnessed a heartbroken family. They were about to lose their father on this earth, and they were not sure of his eternal destiny. I could see and hear their pain; it was devastating. When Chaplain Ron assured them that their dad was at peace with God, the pain eased from their tired faces. They were full of hope and joy because they believed they would one day meet their father in heaven.

Never again did I doubt why Medicare required a chaplain. From that day forward, it did not matter if only one patient in a million needed a chaplain. If one soul is saved by learning about God's loving grace, it is worth every penny.

What would have been a devastating death turned out to be a celebration of victory through Christ. The family asked Chaplain Ron to officiate the funeral along with their family pastor. The service was a beautiful home-going celebration. The patient's daughters became hospice volunteers for our agency, and they stayed in touch for many years.

Words For Thought From Chaplain Ron

God loves each and every one of us and has given us the chance while we are still amongst the living to accept Jesus Christ as Lord and Savior of our lives. We all must face a time appointed unto us to transition from this life into the next. By following God's simple plan of salvation, we are assured of the victory over death and an eternal home in heaven. Some have already made this choice, and others thank God while they still have a chance with a change of mind and claim the last blessing of this life.

God's Simple Plan of Salvation

Written by Chaplain Ron

"For all have sinned, and come short of the glory of God."
Romans 3:23

"For the wages of sin *is* death; but the gift of God *is* eternal life through Jesus Christ our Lord."
Romans 6:23

"But God commendeth his love toward us, in that, while we were yet sinners, Christ died for us."
Romans 5:8

"That if thou shalt confess with thy mouth the Lord Jesus, and shalt believe in thine heart that God hath raised him from the dead, thou shalt be saved."
Romans 10:9

"For whosoever shall call upon the name of the Lord shall be saved."
Romans 10:13

Conclusion

It Began at the End

So teach us to number our days, that we may apply our hearts unto wisdom
—*Psalm 90:12*

Written by Michelle and Chaplain Ron

These are just a few of our stories about God's blessings. These stories would not have been possible if it had not been for the life of one woman. At the age of thirty, she suffered from depression and wanted to die. However, her despair gave way to light and over time she found a new purpose for living. Her name was Florence Nightingale, founder of the nursing profession (*https://www/bibliography.com*). She died at the age of ninety after helping countless soldiers and individuals. Some believe that she and those who introduced antiseptics to medicine did more than anyone to help relieve human suffering.

We thank God for the Last Blessing upon Florence Nightingale's life, for her blessing also became God's blessing unto all mankind.

We end with the hymn "Amazing Grace" because grace is a blessing from God that gives us access unto salvation and eternal life through Jesus Christ.

It is true and it is perfect, God's amazing Grace is a blessing.

Amazing Grace

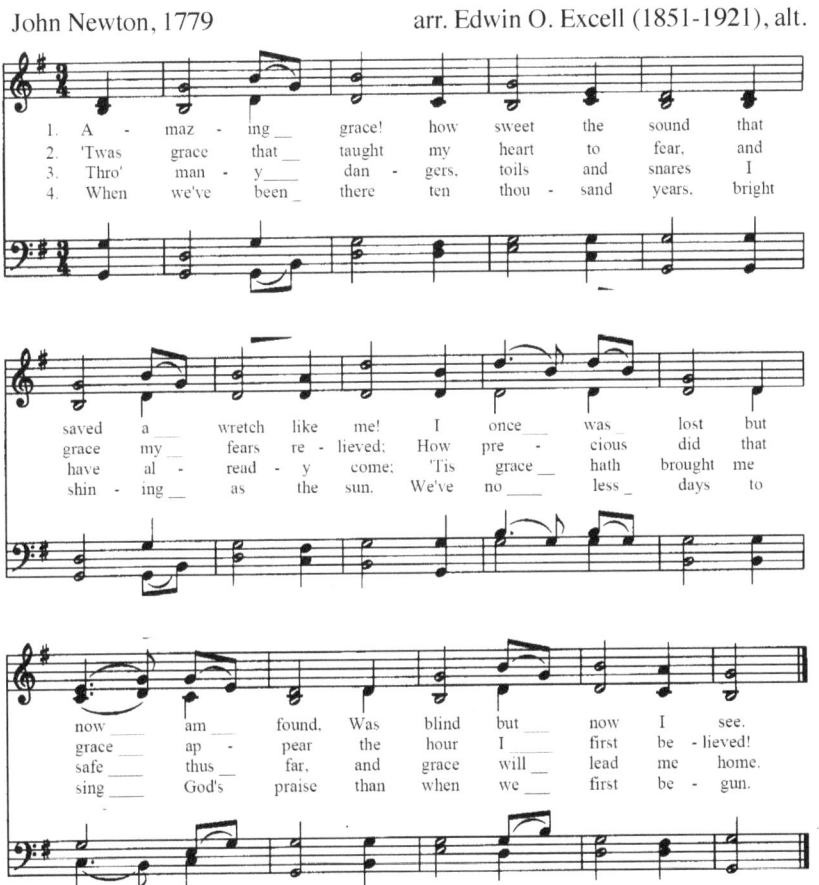

References

"Hope." *Merriam-Webster.com*. Merriam-Webster, n.d. Web. 8 June 2017.
Brungardmd.com/hospice-palliative-medicine/food-water-for-the-journey-at-life's-end

Allowing Prn orders for morphine may result in untimely death for copd patients hospicepatient.org/no-prn-morphine-copd-html

Use of Morphine
Carenotkilling.org.uk/news/use-of-morphine

Managing Nausea and Vomiting
Verywell.com/managing-nausea-and-vomiting-1132089

"PTSD." *Merriam-Webster.com*. Merriam-Webster, n.d. Web. 8 June 2017.

Kübler-Ross model. (2017, May 28). In *Wikipedia, The Free Encyclopedia*. Retrieved

16:02, June 8, 2017, from https://en.wikipedia.org/w/index.php?title=K%C3%BCbler-Ross_model&oldid=782640581.

The 5 Stages of Grief & Loss
Psychcentral.com/lib/the-5-stages-of-loss-and-grief

Alzheimer's Association. (2017). Quick facts. Retrieved from:

http://www.alz.org/facts/overview.asp

Florence Nightingale. Biography. Retrieved from : https://www.biography.com/people/florence-nightingale-9423539

American Hospice Foundation (2017). Retrieved from:

https://americanhospice.org/learning-about-hospice/

"Hospice." *Merriam-Webster.com*. Merriam-Webster, n.d. Web. 10 Aug. 2017.

Resources

Agencies and Associations

Alzheimer's Association
www.alz.org
(800) 272-3900
American Cancer Society
www.cancer.org
Help line - (800) 227-2345
American Heart Association

www.heart.org
1-800-242-8721

Center for Disease Control
www.cdc.gov
(800) 232-4636

Meals on Wheels Association of America
www.mowaa.org
(730) 548-8024

National Hospice and Palliative Care Organization
www.nhpco.org
(703) 837-1500

U.S. Dept. of Veteran Affairs
www.va.gov
Crisis Line – (800) 273-8255

Bereavement, Grief, Death and Dying

AARP
www.aarp.org
1-888-687-2277
Caring Connections
www.caringinfo.org
(800) 658-8898

About the Authors

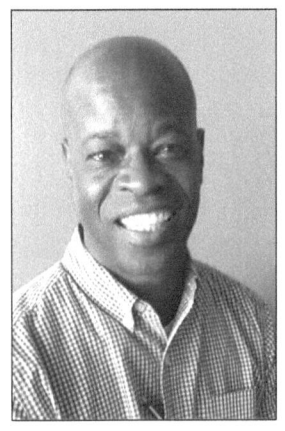

Ronald Lewis has been working in Hospice Care for over twelve years. He has served in the roles of Chaplain, Bereavement Coordinator, Community Outreach Coordinator, and Director of Spiritual and Community Services. Ron is also certified in dementia care and holds a B.S. degree from Lancaster Bible College and a Master's Degree in Christian Counseling Psychology from Southwest Seminary. Chaplain Ron, is actively involved and supports the National Alzheimer's Association and American Cancer Society. He is married with two children and one grandchild. His favorite scripture is Psalm 1, and his favorite hymn is "How Great thou Art."

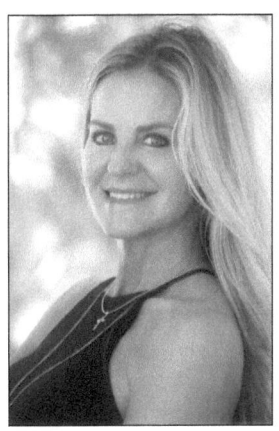

Michelle Poston is a Registered Nurse and has worked in hospice for twelve years. She gives God credit for her nursing degree and nursing career. The bulk of her career has been hospice and wound care. She loves the beach and is happy to call Myrtle Beach home. She thanks God for her wonderful family and circle of friends. The love of her life is her two children and two granddaughters. She happily waits for October 2017 and God's blessing of a new grandbaby boy. Michelle actively supports the Tara Hall Home for Boys in Georgetown, SC and the homeless shelters in Myrtle Beach, SC. Her favorite verse is Proverbs 14:31 and her favorite hymn is "The Old Rugged Cross."

Ron and Michelle have worked together on thousands of care cases over the course of their careers. God has blessed them with the ability to help patients and their loved ones during the most difficult time in their lives. They believe God brought them together twelve years ago for a purpose.